Standards of Emergency Nursing Practice

EMERGENCY NURSES ASSOCIATION

STANDARDS OF EMERGENCY NURSING PRACTICE

THIRD EDITION

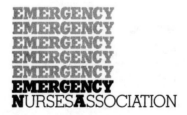

THESE STANDARDS OF EMERGENCY NURSING PRACTICE
ARE ACKNOWLEDGED BY THE AMERICAN NURSES ASSOCIATION

Senior Vice President and Publisher: Alison Miller
Editor-in-Chief: Nancy Coon
Editor: Robin Carter
Assistant Editor: Kerri Rabbitt
Project Manager: Patricia Tannian
Production Editor: Ann E. Rogers
Designer: Cheryl Gelfand-Grant
Cover Designer: Teresa Breckwoldt
Manufacturing Supervisor: Betty Richmond

THIRD EDITION
Copyright © 1995 by Mosby–Year Book, Inc.

Previous editions copyrighted 1983, 1991

Printed in the United States of America
Composition by Mosby Electronic Production, St. Louis
Printing/binding by Plus Communications, Inc.

Mosby–Year Book, Inc.
11830 Westline Industrial Drive
St. Louis, Missouri 63146

Library of Congress Cataloging in Publication Data

Emergency Nurses Association.
  Standards of emergency nursing practice / Emergency Nurses
    Association.—3rd ed.
      p. cm.
  Includes bibliographical references.
  ISBN 0-8151-3048-1
  1. Emergency nursing—Standards. I. Title.
  [DNLM: 1. Emergency Nursing—standards—United States. 2. Nursing
    Care—standards—United States. WY 154 E52075s 1994]
  RT120.E4E45 1994a
  610.73'61—dc20
  DNLM/DLC
  for Library of Congress   94-9563
                                                                     CIP

94 95 96 97 98 / 9 8 7 6 5 4 3 2 1

Acknowledgments

Third Edition

LEAD EDITOR

Nancy Stephens Donatelli, RN, MS, CEN, CNA
Director: Outpatient & Senior Services
The Medical Center
Beaver, PA

EDITORS

Laurie Flaherty, RN, MS, CEN
Clinical Educator: Emergency Department
Georgetown University Hospital
Washington, DC

Linda Greenberg, RN, MS, CEN
Director: Emergency, Trauma, Air Ambulance Services
Sacred Heart Medical Center
Spokane, WA

Linda Larson, RN, PhD(c), FNP, CEN
Nurse Practitioner
G.K. Deagman, MD, PC
Aurora, CO

Lorene Newberry, RN, MS, CEN
Clinical Nurse Specialist: Emergency Center
Kennestone Hospital in Marietta
Marietta, GA

ENA Staff Liaisons

Eleanore Kirsch, RN, MS, CEN
Deputy Executive Director

Luanne Lenick
Coordinator: Professional Services

Nancy Stonis, RN, BSN
Director: Professional Services

Authors

Second Edition

Eileen Alexander, RN, MSN, CEN

Joyce Dains, RN, DrPH

Joanne Ingalls McKay, RN, MSN, CEN

Kathy Jordan, RN, MS, CS, CCRN, CEN

Nancy Lyle, RN, MSN

Marilyn Rice, RN, BSN, MPA, CEN

Jill Schoerger Walsh, RN, MS

First Edition

Pamela W. Bourg, RN, MS

Susan Budassi Sheehy, RN, MSN, CEN

Virginia Curtin Capasso, RN, MSN

Joyce Dains, RN, MSN

Gail Pisarcik Lenehan, RN, MS, CS

Marguerite T. Littleton, RN, MSN

Judy Spinella, RN, MS

Contents

Preface

The third edition of *Standards of Emergency Nursing Practice (Standards)* was revised in 1993 as part of the cyclical revision process of all Emergency Nurses Association (ENA) documents. Those familiar with the second edition will note the change in size of this edition. Also, in an effort to streamline *Standards*, make it more user friendly, and prevent readers from identifying the resources as standards rather than suggested formats, the resources have been removed from the text of *Standards* and are now referenced at the back of this document. ENA has developed numerous other resources such as *Triage: Meeting the Challenge, Emergency Clinical Nurse Specialist Guidelines, Emergency Nurses Guide to Nursing Diagnosis, Emergency Department Patient Classification Systems Manual, Orientation to Emergency Nursing: Diversity in Practice, Pediatric Emergency Resource Guide,* and *Resource Document for Nursing Care of the Trauma Patient.* These new publications provide comprehensive information on their respective subjects, including data covered by the resource documents in the second edition of *Standards.*

Agencies or individuals who consult this document should understand that these standards represent the philosophy of the Emergency Nurses Association. The standards presented constitute recommended goals and general guidelines of care, education, and experience levels for emergency nurses. The standards do not constitute a legal or regulatory document.

Readers are directed to utilize this Preface and the Introduction to enhance understanding of specific terms used in *Standards*, including the "competent" and "excellent" levels.

It should be noted that the term "emergency nurse" throughout the document designates a registered professional nurse licensed to practice nursing.

EMERGENCY
EMERGENCY
EMERGENCY
EMERGENCY
EMERGENCY
EMERGENCY
NURSESASSOCIATION

INTRODUCTION

HISTORY OF ENA STANDARDS DEVELOPMENT

The original standards were developed in 1983. The concepts of professionalism, research, education, and practice provided the cornerstone for the development of those standards. The original authors, in concert with ENA leadership, transformed their vision for emergency nursing practice into the philosophy and standards that guided the development of the profession.

The first revision process, completed in 1990, expanded and further defined the original framework and clarified the distinction between competence and excellence, focusing on measurable professional behaviors of the emergency nurse.

RECENT CHANGES IN THE HEALTH CARE ENVIRONMENT THAT AFFECT STANDARDS DEVELOPMENT

The nursing profession is integral to the continuing examination and development of a more cost-effective and efficient health care system. One aspect of nursing's contribution to health care reform is the standards by which the quality of practice, service, and education can be measured.

At present, the health care system is being closely scrutinized. Previously accepted patterns of health care utilization, reimbursement, and treatment are being reexamined. Many organizations and government agencies are involved in the initiative to improve the effectiveness and efficiency of health care. Among these are the American Nurses Association (ANA), the Agency for Health Care Policy and Research (AHCPR), the Joint Commission on the Accreditation of Healthcare Organizations (JCAHO), private insurers, various health care organizations, and other private and government agencies.

AHCPR is responsible for developing guidelines that will direct clinical practice by providing links between diagnosis, treatments, and outcomes, and by describing the alternatives available for each patient. These guidelines, developed by multidisciplinary teams, will serve as frameworks for decision trees that will enable both consumers and providers to make informed treatment choices.

JCAHO requires hospitals to set standards of patient care with measurable clinical outcomes. JCAHO defines patient care standards as nursing or medical diagnoses that are directed toward achieving specific patient outcomes.

Professional nursing organizations have developed guidelines and standards that address the nursing care of patients. One of the issues in the development of standards is the lack of consistent terminology. As previously noted, the terms "standards of care," "standards of practice," and "guidelines" have different mean-

4

ings for different groups. The issue is further complicated by variability in focus and practical application. In this revision, ENA has addressed the issue of inconsistent terminology by adapting the format used in the ANA *Standards of Clinical Nursing Practice.*

PRESENTATION OF THE 1994 STANDARDS

The ENA endorsed the 1991 *ANA Standards of Clinical Nursing Practice* as generic nursing standards. These standards apply to care that is provided to all patients by registered nurses engaged in clinical practice, regardless of clinical specialty, practice setting, or educational preparation (ANA, 1991). These standards of practice are the basis of nursing practice and cannot be subsumed or delegated to individuals not licensed to practice professional nursing. The *ANA Standards of Clinical Nursing Practice* includes standards of care and standards of professional performance.

STANDARDS OF CARE

- Assessment
- Diagnosis
- Outcome Identification
- Planning
- Implementation
- Evaluation

STANDARDS OF PROFESSIONAL PERFORMANCE

- Quality of Care
- Performance Appraisal
- Education
- Collegiality
- Ethics
- Collaboration
- Research
- Resource Utilization

In the third edition of the ENA *Standards,* the ANA generic standards have been adapted as the basis for the further development of emergency nursing specialty standards. This has been done to facilitate the unification of nursing standards and requisite nomenclature. ENA has added a triage standard of care to the ANA listing because it is specific to the practice of emergency nursing. ENA also recognizes that there are different terms being used in the health care environment to refer to the people served (e.g., patient, client, consumer, customer). ENA has chosen to refer to those served by emergency nurses as "patients."

A standard is an acknowledged measure of quantitative or qualitative value and is designed to set forth a combination of skills, education, and performance, which a nurse should strive to achieve. The generic standards apply to all nurses in all settings, whereas the specialty standards apply to all nurses practicing in an emergency care setting. The standards are not designed as a legal model to dictate whether an emergency nurse is competent or excellent.

The competent level in each standard identifies the levels of performance the emergency nurse, or an institution, should consider in establishing goals for the nurse's professional practice. Each area set forth in the standards does not necessarily have to be met for the nurse's performance to be competent. Competent emergency nursing is demonstrated by sound clinical judgment in autonomous practice. Emergency nursing at the excellent level is practice that surpasses the competent level and contributes to the growth of emergency nursing practice. It is important to remember when evaluating competence or excellence that total performance should be evaluated over time and in relation to specific events and individual environments. ENA has taken the position that entry level into practice should be at the baccalaureate level. ENA also believes that participation in the professional organization is a key factor in the development of professional nurses.

The ENA Standards of Care apply to all types of patients and all age-groups. The ENA Standards of Professional Performance apply to all clinicians, including clinical nurses, nurse educators, advanced practice nurses, and nurses practicing in a management role.

The following is the format for this revision of the *Standards*:

- Statement of generic standard
- Statement of specialty standard
- Rationale for specialty standard
- Statement of generic measurement criteria
- Statement of specialty measurement criteria at the competent and excellent levels

Criteria including key indicators of competent and excellent practice will be revised on a cyclical basis to incorporate advances in scientific knowledge, clinical practice, and technology (ENA, 1991).

SUMMARY

Since 1983, the *Standards* have been a springboard for growth within a dynamic emergency nursing environment. As such, they continue to be used for a variety of purposes:

- Criteria-based job descriptions
- Criteria-based performance evaluations
- Department policies and procedures
- Standardized emergency care plans
- Interviewing and hiring practices for emergency nurses
- Development of orientation, in-service, and continuing education programs
- Creation and revision of emergency care forms
- Quality improvement programs and activities
- Development of curricula for baccalaureate and graduate emergency nursing programs
- Integration of standards and guidelines into the blueprint for the Certification Examination for Emergency Nurses.
- Resource document for a variety of other ENA publications

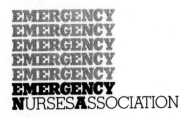

STANDARDS OF CARE

The following section delineates the ENA Standards of Care, which include:

The format of each subsection includes generic standards and specialty standards. The generic standards and measurement criteria were published by ANA in *Standards of Clinical Nursing Practice* (ANA, 1991) and are applicable to all nurses.

The specialty standards and measurement criteria are derivations of the generic standards and criteria. They specifically define how an emergency nurse should perform at the competent and excellent levels.

Comprehensive Standard I   Assessment

Generic Standard The nurse collects client health data.

Specialty Standard The emergency nurse initiates accurate and ongoing assessment of physical, psychological, and social problems of patients within the emergency care system.

Rationale Assessment is a series of systematic, organized, and deliberate actions to identify and obtain data about the patient. This assessment provides the data base for determination of state of health or illness of the patient.

GENERIC MEASUREMENT CRITERIA

1. The priority of data collection is determined by the client's immediate condition or needs.
2. Pertinent data are collected using appropriate assessment techniques.
3. Data collection involves the client, significant others, and health care providers when appropriate.
4. The data collection process is systematic and ongoing.
5. Relevant data are documented in a retrievable form.

SPECIALTY MEASUREMENT CRITERIA

1. Systematic and pertinent collection of data about health status of every patient is assessed.

   Competent Level
   - Obtains initial focused subjective and objective data through history taking, physical examination, review of records, and communication with health care providers, significant others, and caretakers, as appropriate.
   - Conducts assessment within the framework of holistic professional nursing practice.
   - Performs the initial assessment based on triage acuity. Ongoing assessments are performed as established by department policies, and as warranted by patient response.
   - Uses assessment techniques and criteria that are pertinent to the patient's age-specific physical, psychological, and social needs.
   - Records relevant data for every patient in a retrievable form, as appropriate to the nature and severity of illness or injury.
   - Communicates significant data to appropriate personnel throughout the patient's emergency care experience.

Excellent Level

- Obtains initial and comprehensive subjective and objective data through history taking, physical examination, review of records, and communication with health care providers, significant others, and caretakers as appropriate.
- Serves as a role model and resource person to facilitate the performance of accurate and ongoing nursing assessments.
- Identifies nursing or system deficiencies that may impede adequate assessment.
- Participates in development and implementation of tools, systems, and techniques that enhance nursing assessment and documentation.

Comprehensive Standard II   Diagnosis

Generic Standard The nurse analyzes assessment data in determining diagnoses.

Specialty Standard The emergency nurse analyzes assessment data to formulate nursing diagnoses and identify collaborative problems for each patient.

Rationale Use of diagnostic reasoning in the analysis of assessment data helps determine the patient's health status.

GENERIC MEASUREMENT CRITERIA

1. Diagnoses are derived from the assessment data.
2. Diagnoses are validated with the client, significant others, and other health care providers, when possible.
3. Diagnoses are documented in a manner that facilitates the determination of expected outcomes and plan of care.

SPECIALTY MEASUREMENT CRITERIA

1. For every patient, the emergency nurse identifies the actual and high-risk health problems or diagnoses based on pertinent data collected in the focused assessment.

Competent Level

- Identifies nursing diagnoses and/or collaborative problems, based on defining characteristics, that is, signs and symptoms recognized during a focused, systematic assessment.
- Utilizes assessment data from pertinent sources to identify collaborative problems and formulate nursing diagnoses.
- Communicates and validates nursing diagnoses with other health care providers as appropriate.
- Identifies and communicates collaborative problems to other health care providers as appropriate.
- Formulates nursing diagnoses consistent with current knowledge that is research based.
- Documents nursing diagnoses and/or collaborative problems on each patient in a retrievable form.

Excellent Level

- Anticipates and recognizes nursing diagnoses and/or collaborative problems, based on atypical or subtle defining characteristics.
- Acts as role model and resource person to facilitate and validate the analysis of assessment data for accurate and appropriate identification of nursing diagnoses and/or collaborative problems.
- Identifies nursing and system deficiencies that may impede adequate identification of nursing diagnoses and/or collaborative problems.
- Participates in the development and implementation of tools and systems to facilitate effective use of nursing diagnoses.
- Clinically tests nursing diagnoses in emergency nursing for appropriateness and relevance.
- Validates nursing diagnoses for specific emergency patients and patient populations.
- Participates in development of nursing diagnoses to expand the current body of knowledge regarding the care of emergency patients.

Comprehensive Standard III   Outcome Identification

Generic Standard The nurse identifies expected outcomes individualized to the client.

Specialty Standard The emergency nurse identifies expected outcomes individualized to the emergency patient based on assessment and nursing diagnoses and/or collaborative problems.

Rationale Outcome identification is the bridge from assessment and nursing diagnoses to intervention and evaluation, providing focus and clarity to the plan of care.

GENERIC MEASUREMENT CRITERIA

1. Outcomes are derived from the diagnoses.
2. Outcomes are documented as measurable goals.
3. Outcomes are mutually formulated with the client and other health care providers, when possible.
4. Outcomes are realistic in relation to the client's present and potential capabilities.
5. Outcomes are attainable in relation to resources available to the client.
6. Outcomes include a time estimate for attainment.
7. Outcomes provide direction for continuity of care.

SPECIALTY MEASUREMENT CRITERIA

1. Physical, psychological, and emotional outcomes are identified for each patient as appropriate.

Competent Level
- Identifies measurable short-term and long-term outcomes.
- Identifies appropriate time frames for attainment of outcomes related to patient's nursing diagnoses and/or collaborative problems.
- Communicates expected outcomes to other health care providers to ensure continuity of care.

Excellent Level
- Acts as a resource for the development of an outcome-driven plan of care for each patient.
- Develops peer education that emphasizes identification and utilization of patient outcome measures.
- Develops guidelines or clinical and/or critical pathways of expected outcomes for groups of patients with similar diagnoses and/or collaborative problems.

Generic Standard The nurse develops a plan of care that prescribes interventions to attain expected outcomes.

Specialty Standard The emergency nurse formulates a plan of care for the emergency patient based on assessment, nursing diagnoses and/or collaborative problems, and outcome identification.

Rationale Safe, effective emergency patient care results from active, focused planning by the emergency nurse.

GENERIC MEASUREMENT CRITERIA

1. The plan is individualized to the client's condition or needs.
2. The plan is developed with the client, significant others, and health care providers, when appropriate.
3. The plan reflects current nursing practice.
4. The plan is documented.
5. The plan provides for continuity of care.

SPECIALTY MEASUREMENT CRITERIA

1. The plan of care for the emergency patient is systematic and consistent with safe, effective patient care.

Competent Level
- Develops a plan of care for each patient based on current scientific knowledge.
- Collaborates with significant others and appropriate heath care providers in developing the plan of care.
- Identifies priorities for nursing actions, patient goals, and patient outcomes.
- Addresses environmental, physical, and psychological stressors in the plan of care.
- Incorporates teaching and learning principles in the plan of care.
- Communicates plan of care to other health care providers to ensure continuity of care.

Excellent Level
- Develops, implements, and evaluates guidelines for patient care.
- Acts as a resource for the use of guidelines for patient care.
- Participates in the development, implementation, and evaluation of tools to facilitate planning care, such as guidelines or clinical and/or critical pathways.
- Designs departmental framework to facilitate involvement of patient and significant others in plan of care.
- Develops plan of care that addresses high-risk nursing diagnoses and/or collaborative problems.
- Develops plan of care that recognizes implications of patient's long-term problems.

Comprehensive Standard V   Implementation

Generic Standard   The nurse implements the interventions identified in the plan of care.

Specialty Standard   The emergency nurse implements a plan of care based on assessment, nursing diagnoses and/or collaborative problems, and outcome identification.

Rationale   Assessment data, nursing diagnoses and/or collaborative problems, outcome criteria, and planning provide a foundation for implementation of requisite interventions.

GENERIC MEASUREMENT CRITERIA

1. Interventions are consistent with the established plan of care.
2. Interventions are implemented in a safe and appropriate manner.
3. Interventions are documented.

SPECIALTY MEASUREMENT CRITERIA

1. Interventions are based on priority of patient need and consideration of significant others.

Competent Level

-   Implements plan of care for each patient.
-   Performs appropriate patient monitoring.
-   Provides requisite education for patient and significant others.
-   Anticipates need for additional resources to implement interventions.
-   Works collaboratively with other health care providers, as appropriate, to implement interventions.

Excellent Level

-   Identifies and independently performs comprehensive interventions.
-   Works collaboratively with other health care providers, as appropriate, to implement more complex interventions.

Comprehensive Standard VI   Evaluation

Generic Standard The nurse evaluates the client's progress toward attainment of outcomes.

Specialty Standard The emergency nurse evaluates and modifies the plan of care based on observable patient responses and attainment of expected outcomes.

Rationale The dynamic nature of emergency patient care requires continual evaluation to optimize achievement of patient outcomes.

GENERIC MEASUREMENT CRITERIA

1. Evaluation is systematic and ongoing.
2. The client's responses to interventions are documented.
3. The effectiveness of interventions is evaluated in relation to outcomes.
4. Ongoing assessment data are used to revise diagnoses, outcomes, and the plan of care, as needed.
5. Revisions in diagnoses, outcomes, and the plan of care are documented.
6. The client, significant others, and health care providers are involved in the evaluation process, when appropriate.

SPECIALTY MEASUREMENT CRITERIA

1. The patient's response to interventions is continually evaluated to determine progress toward resolution of immediate needs.

    ## Competent Level
    - Utilizes current patient data to measure progress toward attainment of patient outcomes.
    - Utilizes data from the patient, significant others, and other health care providers to evaluate patient responses to intervention.
    - Documents patient's response to interventions and changes in patient's condition, and revises the plan of care as appropriate.
    - Evaluates progress toward achievement of expected outcomes, modifying interventions and/or outcomes as appropriate.
    - Modifies outcomes as needed when changes occur in patient abilities and available resources.

    ## Excellent Level
    - Acts as a role model for comprehensive evaluation of patient care.
    - Functions as a resource person for evaluation of patient care.

Generic Standard None

Specialty Standard The emergency nurse triages each patient and determines priority of care based on physical, psychological, and social needs, as well as factors influencing patient flow through the emergency care system.*

Rationale Triage facilitates the flow of patients through the emergency care system to ensure timely evaluation of patient needs and to address spatial, temporal, and administrative demands on the system.

GENERIC MEASUREMENT CRITERIA None

---

*ENA believes that safe, effective, and efficient triage can be performed only by a registered professional nurse educated in the principles of triage with a minimum of 6 months' experience in emergency nursing.

SPECIALTY MEASUREMENT CRITERIA

1. Assessment
   A rapid, systematic collection of data relevant to each patient's chief complaint, age, and social situation is conducted to obtain sufficient information to determine patient acuity and any immediate physical, psychological, or social needs.

   ## Competent Level

   - Performs focused assessment of chief complaint on each patient entering the emergency care system, collecting subjective and objective data.
   - Assesses patients in a timely manner according to established triage criteria.
   - Documents triage assessment, including appropriate subjective and objective data.

   ## Excellent Level

   - Serves as a role model and resource person in the assessment phase of triage.
   - Participates in development, implementation, and/or revision of triage assessment systems such as age-specific guidelines and complaint-specific protocols.
   - Participates in development, implementation, and/or revision of tools for documenting triage assessment.

2. Diagnosis
   Information gathered in the assessment phase is analyzed to determine the severity of physical, psychological, social, and educational needs.

Competent Level

- Differentiates severity of patient problems.
- Identifies nursing diagnoses and/or collaborative problems when possible.
- Documents clinical impressions.

Excellent Level

- Recognizes nursing diagnoses and/or collaborative problems using atypical or subtle defining characteristics.
- Acts as role model and resource person for triage confirmation, identification of collaborative problems, and/or validation of nursing diagnoses.

3. Outcome Identification
   Individualized expected outcomes are identified for each patient.

Competent Level

- Formulates outcomes relative to nursing diagnoses and/or collaborative problems, available resources, patient abilities, and input.
- Identifies and documents measurable criteria such as time estimate and objective data.

Excellent Level

- Addresses atypical presentations to identify high risk outcomes.
- Acts as a role model and resource person for confirmation and validation of outcome identification.

4. Planning

    The urgency of physical, psychological, social, and educational needs is determined, and the course of action is formulated to attain expected outcomes.

    ### Competent Level

    - Differentiates urgency of patient problems and prioritizes care, assigning the patient to the appropriate acuity level.
    - Directs the patient to the appropriate treatment area, based on assessment, diagnoses, outcome identification, and acuity level.
    - Communicates pertinent information to other health care providers.
    - Documents acuity and individual plan of care.
    - Identifies interventions to attain expected outcomes.

    ### Excellent Level

    - Anticipates patient needs and interventions, based on identification of actual and high-risk health problems.
    - Acts as a role model and resource person for the planning phase of triage.

5. Implementation
   Interventions are implemented as identified in the plan of care.

Competent Level

- Initiates independent nursing measures.
- Initiates diagnostic procedures per established triage protocols.
- Initiates treatment per established protocols, for example, antipyretics.
- Documents all interventions.
- Communicates pertinent information to patient and significant others.
- Mobilizes additional resources as needed.

Excellent Level

- Participates in development and implementation of independent nursing measures and collaborative protocols.
- Identifies implementation practices requiring revision or change.
- Acts as role model and resource person for independent and collaborative interventions.

6. Evaluation
   The patient's response to intervention is evaluated.

Competent Level

- Reassesses the patient according to acuity and established procedures.
- Evaluates and documents the effectiveness of all interventions as appropriate.
- Revises the plan of care, acuity level, and the expected outcome based on new information or changes in assessment data.

Excellent Level

- Acts as a role model and resource person for the evaluation phase of the triage process.
- Identifies nursing or system deficiencies that may impede adequate patient evaluation.

EMERGENCY
EMERGENCY
EMERGENCY
EMERGENCY
EMERGENCY
EMERGENCY
NURSES**A**SSOCIATION

STANDARDS
OF PROFESSIONAL
PERFORMANCE

The following section delineates the ENA Standards of Professional Performance, which include:

The format of each subsection includes generic standards and specialty standards. The generic standards and measurement criteria are published by ANA in *Standards of Clinical Nursing Practice* (ANA, 1991) and are applicable to all nurses.

The specialty standards and measurement criteria are derivations of the generic standards and criteria. They specifically define how an emergency nurse should perform at the competent and excellent levels.

Comprehensive Standard VIII   Quality of Care

Generic Standard The nurse systematically evaluates the quality and effectiveness of nursing practice.

Specialty Standard The emergency nurse evaluates the quality and effectiveness of emergency nursing practice.

Rationale Evaluation of emergency nursing practice is concurrent and retrospective to ensure that the quality of care is maintained.

GENERIC MEASUREMENT CRITERIA

1. The nurse participates in quality of care activities as appropriate to the individual's position, education, and practice environment. Such activities may include:

   - Identification of aspects of care that are important for quality monitoring.
   - Identification of indicators used to monitor quality and effectiveness of nursing care.
   - Collection of data to monitor quality and effectiveness of nursing care.
   - Analysis of quality data to identify opportunities for improving care.
   - Formulation of recommendations to improve nursing practice or client outcomes.
   - Implementation of activities to enhance the quality of nursing practice.
   - Participation on interdisciplinary teams that evaluate clinical practice or health services.
   - Development of policies and procedures to improve quality of care.

2. The nurse uses the results of quality of care activities to initiate changes in practice.
3. The nurse uses the results of quality of care activities to initiate changes throughout the health care delivery system, as appropriate.

SPECIALTY MEASUREMENT CRITERIA

1. The emergency nurse develops and implements a comprehensive plan for assessing and improving the quality of care for emergency patients.

Competent Level

- Participates in the development and implementation of the plan for assessing and improving quality of care for emergency patients.
- Participates in the development and implementation of actions, resolutions, and ongoing monitoring activities designed to improve emergency nursing practice and the health care system.
- Communicates and documents quality of care concerns that are identified individually as well as through peer review.

Excellent Level

- Works collaboratively to develop, implement, and evaluate a multidisciplinary quality assessment and improvement plan.
- Implements and evaluates actions, resolutions, and ongoing indicators designed to improve emergency nursing practice.
- Develops, implements, and evaluates quality of care actions to monitor indicators for triage excellence.
- Develops, implements, and evaluates methods to enhance the quality of nursing care.
- Initiates mechanisms to address quality of care concerns.
- Monitors regulatory and legislative activities that affect the quality of emergency nursing practice.
- Participates in collaborative quality assessment and improvement studies.

2. The emergency nurse continually assesses and evaluates the care delivery system using quality improvement principles and practices.

Competent Level

- Identifies internal and external customers, including patients, physicians, staff, other departments, and community agencies.
- Assesses customer needs to maximize customer satisfaction.
- Collaborates with other departments to improve and enhance patient care delivery on a continual basis.
- Participates in system analysis and redesign to increase efficiency and productivity.

Excellent Level

- Acts as a resource on quality improvement principles and methods.
- Develops customer satisfaction surveys.
- Initiates and leads multidisciplinary quality action teams.
- Develops, implements, and evaluates system analysis plans to increase efficiency and productivity.

Comprehensive Standard IX   Performance Appraisal

Generic Standard The nurse evaluates his or her own nursing practice in relation to professional practice standards and relevant statutes and regulations.

Specialty Standard The emergency nurse adheres to established standards of practice, including activities and behaviors that characterize professional status.

Rationale Safe and effective nursing practice depends on application of a specific body of knowledge and skills congruent with professional behavior.

GENERIC MEASUREMENT CRITERIA

1. The nurse engages in performance appraisal on a regular basis, identifying areas of strength as well as areas for professional and practice development.
2. The nurse seeks constructive feedback regarding his or her own practice.
3. The nurse takes action to achieve goals identified during performance appraisal.
4. The nurse participates in peer review as appropriate.

SPECIALTY MEASUREMENT CRITERIA

1. The emergency nurse is accountable for his or her actions.

Competent Level

- Assumes responsibility for his or her actions.
- Possesses a knowledge base related to:
  - Collection and processing of data related to physical, psychological, and social needs of noncritical and critical status patients.
  - Identification of nursing diagnoses.
  - Outcome identification.
  - Development of a comprehensive plan for nursing care.
  - Implementation of a plan of nursing care.
  - Evaluation of care based on observable responses.
- Understands regulatory and legislative issues that affect the practice of emergency nursing.

Excellent Level

- Utilizes authority and responsibility to provide competency-based job descriptions and nursing performance reviews.
- Monitors regulatory and legislative activities that affect the practice of the emergency nurse and utilizes those key issues as a part of the performance appraisal process.

2. The emergency nurse participates in clinical and peer review to evaluate practice.

Competent Level

- Uses self-evaluation, peer evaluation, and feedback from supervisors and patients to modify and enhance practice.

Excellent Level

- Plans, initiates, and evaluates clinical care and the peer review process to assess professional practice.
- Develops, implements, and evaluates programs of competency-based performance appraisal.

Comprehensive Standard X Education

Generic Standard The nurse acquires and maintains current knowledge in nursing practice.

Specialty Standard The emergency nurse recognizes self-learning needs and is accountable for maximizing professional development and optimal emergency nursing practice.

Rationale Inherent in the process of continuing education is the responsibility for self-learning and integration of that learning into daily practice.

GENERIC MEASUREMENT CRITERIA

1. The nurse participates in ongoing educational activities related to clinical knowledge and professional issues.
2. The nurse seeks experiences to maintain clinical skills.
3. The nurse seeks knowledge and skills appropriate to the practice setting.

SPECIALTY MEASUREMENT CRITERIA

1. The emergency nurse is responsible for acquiring and demonstrating attainment of a defined body of emergency nursing knowledge.

Competent Level
- Completes appropriate orientation to the emergency care area.
- Demonstrates requisite knowledge and skills for stabilization of the emergency patient.
- Attains BLS provider status.
- Attains ALS and/or PALS provider status as appropriate.
- Attains Certification in Emergency Nursing (CEN®) (strongly recommended).
- Attains TNCC Provider status (minimum level of education for emergency nurses caring for trauma patients).
- Attains ENPC Provider status (recommended for emergency nurses caring for pediatric patients).
- Acts as a clinical preceptor for students and orientees.

Excellent Level
- Serves as a role model for clinical preceptors.
- Acts as a resource person for clinical preceptors.
- Provides continuing education related to the specialty of emergency nursing.
- Contributes relevant information to the literature.
- Continues formal education.
- Attains ALS and/or PALS Instructor status (recommended).
- Attains TNCC instructor status (recommended).
- Attains ENPC instructor status (recommended).
- Develops, implements, monitors, and evaluates competency-based staff education.
- Coordinates and directs preceptor programs.

2. The emergency nurse obtains ongoing education consistent with the role and area of practice.

Competent Level

- Determines professional learning needs and identifies short- and long-term educational goals relevant to his or her own practice.
- Plans activities to achieve educational goals.
- Implements activities to achieve educational goals.
- Shares newly gained knowledge from relevant educational programs with peers.
- Applies knowledge and skills learned through continuing education to improve clinical practice.

Excellent Level

- Exceeds educational activities necessary to meet minimal institutional requirements or requirements for relicensure.
- Recommends practice or system changes based on analysis of information obtained from continuing self-education.
- Coordinates the implementation of changes in department procedures or the care delivery system.

Comprehensive Standard XI Collegiality

Generic Standard The nurse contributes to the professional development of peers, colleagues, and others.

Specialty Standard The emergency nurse engages in activities and behaviors that characterize a professional.

Rationale To promote nursing as a profession and emergency nursing as a specialty, the emergency nurse identifies and demonstrates behaviors congruent with professional status.

GENERIC MEASUREMENT CRITERIA

1. The nurse shares knowledge and skills with colleagues and others.
2. The nurse provides peers with constructive feedback regarding their practice.
3. The nurse contributes to an environment that is conducive to clinical education of nursing students, as appropriate.

SPECIALTY MEASUREMENT CRITERIA

1. The emergency nurse supports the professional development of nursing by promoting understanding of nursing roles and responsibilities.

   ### Competent Level
   - Identifies self and responsibilities to patients and significant others.
   - Identifies self to colleagues and other health care providers.
   - Exercises authority through collegial relationships to maximize department operations and patient outcomes.

   ### Excellent Level
   - Assumes leadership responsibilities in ENA.
   - Participates as a professional nurse in community activities.

2. The emergency nurse is knowledgeable of actual and potential legislation and regulations related to emergency care and the practice of emergency nursing.

Competent Level

- Pursues knowledge of actual and potential regulations and legislation related to health care issues.
- Articulates position to those who affect emergency care legislation and regulation.

Excellent Level

- Participates in activities to promote internal regulation of the profession and autonomous practice.
- Monitors legislative activities that affect emergency nursing practice and emergency care issues.

3. The emergency nurse fosters a professional image of nursing.

Competent Level

- Demonstrates a professional image to peers, other health care providers, the media, and the public.
- Acts as a mentor to potential nurses to encourage entry into nursing.

Excellent Level

- Functions within a leadership role to articulate and demonstrate the professional role of the emergency nurse to peers, other health care providers, the media, and the public.
- Acts as a mentor to nursing peers to encourage professional growth.

4. The emergency nurse has responsibility for public education regarding emergency nursing and the emergency care system.

Competent Level

- Disseminates information concerning access to and use of the emergency care system.

Excellent Level

- Plans and/or participates in community activities to educate consumers about emergency nursing and emergency care.
- Communicates with legislators regarding public policy as it relates to public education and awareness of emergency nursing and emergency care issues.

5. The emergency nurse facilitates learning experiences for peers, other health care providers, students, and volunteers.

Competent Level

- Acts as a teacher, role model, preceptor, and mentor.
- Facilitates the learning of professional nursing students regarding the roles and responsibilities of emergency nurses.
- Educates peers and other health care providers about the roles and responsibilities of the emergency nurse.
- Participates in the orientation of students, peers, volunteers, and other health care providers.
- Participates in the education and, as appropriate, supervision of students and other health care providers during clinical practice.

Excellent Level

- Develops, implements, and evaluates orientation programs, preceptorships, mentoring programs, and education programs related to emergency nursing.
- Participates in the planning, implementation, and evaluation of multidisciplinary educational activities.

Generic Standard The nurse's decisions and actions on behalf of clients are determined in an ethical manner.

Specialty Standard The emergency nurse provides care based on philosophical and ethical concepts. These concepts include reverence for life; respect for the inherent dignity, worth, autonomy, and individuality of each human being; and acknowledging the beliefs of other people.

Rationale The belief in human worth makes up the philosophical foundation on which nursing is based.

GENERIC MEASUREMENT CRITERIA

1. The nurse's practice is guided by the ANA *Code for Nurses.**
2. The nurse maintains patient confidentiality.
3. The nurse acts as a patient advocate.
4. The nurse delivers care in a nonjudgmental and nondiscriminatory manner that is sensitive to patient diversity.
5. The nurse delivers care in a manner that preserves/protects patient autonomy, dignity, and rights.
6. The nurse seeks available resources to help formulate ethical decisions.

---

*American Nurses Association. (1985). *Code for Nurses With Interpretive Statements.* Kansas City, MO: Author.

SPECIALTY MEASUREMENT CRITERIA

1. The emergency nurse provides care that demonstrates ethical beliefs and respect for patient rights.

    ## Competent Level
    - Respects the individuality and human worth of patients regardless of age, sexual orientation, socioeconomic status, cultural or ethnic background, spiritual and ethical beliefs, or the nature of health problems.
    - Respects the dignity, confidentiality, and privacy of patients.

    ## Excellent Level
    - Participates on the institution's ethics committee.
    - Participates in the development and implementation of policies and procedures as they relate to ethical issues in emergency care.
    - Develops, implements, and evaluates programs related to ethical issues in emergency care.
    - Participates in the development and implementation of education to increase community awareness of advanced directives legislation.
    - Acts as a role model for ethical practice.

2. The emergency nurse functions autonomously to the extent that knowledge, skills, and role permit.

Competent Level

- Acts congruently with institutional and professional practice standards and state nurse practice acts.

Excellent Level

- Initiates case and peer review to evaluate autonomous practice.

3. The emergency nurse exercises authority congruent with the state nurse practice act and demonstrates an awareness of local, state, and federal laws that govern the delivery of care.

Competent Level

- Complies with the state nurse practice act, policies and procedures of the institution, and local, state, and federal statutes.
- Coordinates delivery of patient care.
- Informs patients of legal rights as required.
- Obtains informed consent for each patient as appropriate.
- Follows appropriate policies and procedures when a patient is physically restrained or treated on an involuntary basis.
- Maintains patient rights as delineated by advanced directives and durable power-of-attorney.
- Understands and complies with interfacility transfer guidelines as mandated by the Consolidated Omnibus Budget Reconciliation Act of 1986 (COBRA) legislation.
- Utilizes authority and responsibility as the ultimate decision maker on issues regarding emergency nursing, maintaining accountability for this decision making.

Excellent Level

- Assumes leadership roles in clinical and managerial situations.
- Defines standards of emergency nursing practice within the institution and area of practice.
- Participates in the development and education of policies and procedures related to the legal responsibilities of the emergency nurse.
- Implements and evaluates programs related to legal responsibilities in the provision of emergency care.

Comprehensive Standard XIII   Collaboration

Generic Standard The nurse collaborates with the client, significant others, and health care providers in providing client care.

Specialty Standard The emergency nurse ensures open and timely communication with emergency patients, significant others, and other health care providers through professional collaboration.

Rationale Effective communication between the patient, significant other, and other health care providers promotes positive health practices within the institution and the community.

GENERIC MEASUREMENT CRITERIA

1. The nurse communicates with the client, significant others, and health care providers regarding client care and nursing's role in the provision of care.
2. The nurse consults with health care providers for client care, as needed.
3. The nurse makes referrals, including provisions for continuity of care, as needed.

SPECIALTY MEASUREMENT CRITERIA

1. The emergency nurse ensures open communication with the patient and significant others.

Competent Level
- Provides requisite information to the patient and significant others to enhance the decision-making process.

Excellent Level
- Acts as a resource and a role model to promote involvement by the patient and significant others in the decision-making process.

2. The emergency nurse participates in community education related to emergency care.

Competent Level

- Participates in community education related to emergency nursing and emergency care systems.

Excellent Level

- Plans, implements, and evaluates appropriate educational offerings at the community level.
- Utilizes patient outcome data to develop prevention and/or education programs.

3. The emergency nurse utilizes education of the patient and significant others to clarify learning needs and optimize patient outcomes.

Competent Level

- Provides information about the patient's condition to the patient and significant others, as appropriate, in a way that is consistent with their intellectual and emotional abilities.
- Provides explanations about treatments before their initiation whenever possible.
- Involves patients and significant others in the decision-making process related to therapeutic intervention whenever possible.
- Explains or ensures explanation of medications, treatments, self-care, referral, and/or prevention.
- Provides and explains written instructions regarding after care, follow-up, and/or referral.
- Participates in the development of written discharge instructions.
- Assists patients and significant others in the identification of factors that place them "at risk" for illness or injury.
- Explains methods for illness or injury prevention, as appropriate.

Excellent Level

- Initiates development of alternative instructional methods based on research.
- Evaluates patient educational materials.

4. The emergency nurse functions as a facilitator and liaison among health care providers and health care agencies, respecting their limits, abilities, and responsibilities.

Competent Level

- Participates in multidisciplinary patient care conferences.
- Collaborates with other health care providers to make decisions for each patient's care.

Excellent Level

- Participates in professional and community committees related to emergency care issues.
- Communicates with other specialty nursing organizations and other disciplines to address relevant issues.

Comprehensive Standard XIV   Research

Generic Standard The nurse uses research findings in practice.

Specialty Standard The emergency nurse recognizes, values, and utilizes research to enhance the practice of emergency nursing.

Rationale Research is necessary to develop a body of validated nursing knowledge on which emergency nursing practice is based.

GENERIC MEASUREMENT CRITERIA

1. The nurse uses interventions substantiated by research as appropriate to the individual's position, education, and practice environment.
2. The nurse participates in research activities as appropriate to the individual's position, education, and practice environment. Such activities may include:

   • Identification of clinical problems suitable for nursing research.
   • Participation in data collection.
   • Participation in a unit, organization, or community research committee or program.
   • Sharing of research activities with others.
   • Conducting research.
   • Critiquing research for application to practice.
   • Using research findings in the development of policies, procedures, and guidelines for client care.

SPECIALTY MEASUREMENT CRITERIA

1. The emergency nurse uses information from research literature to improve practice.

   ## Competent Level

   - Possesses current knowledge of research in emergency
     nursing.
   - Acts as a patient advocate in the application of research
     findings to clinical practice.
   - Critiques emergency care research.
   - Shares research findings with peers.

   ## Excellent Level

   - Disseminates research findings to peers and colleagues
     through formal channels.
   - Monitors literature for pertinent research for potential
     practice or health care system changes.
   - Develops and implements changes in practice in
     response to research.
   - Develops and implements changes in the health care
     system in response to research.

2. The emergency nurse participates in research to expand the body of validated knowledge related to emergency nursing.

Competent Level

- Collects and records research data for approved projects in emergency care.
- Identifies clinical problems or questions for research related to emergency care.
- Acts as a patient advocate during the collection of research data.

Excellent Level

- Designs and implements independent research projects related to emergency care.
- Acts as a patient advocate through participation on review committees for the protection of human rights.
- Assists peers in identifying clinical problems for research in emergency care.
- Assists peers in designing and implementing research projects in emergency care.
- Incorporates findings of emergency care research into standards of practice for the setting.
- Pursues avenues for funding research.
- Initiates grant proposals for research projects in emergency care.

3. The emergency nurse collaborates with colleagues in other disciplines engaged in research in the practice setting.

Competent Level
- Participates in and supports interdisciplinary research.
- Assists in identification of research subjects.

Excellent Level
- Initiates and facilitates interdisciplinary research.
- Maintains an awareness of current epidemiologic trends and shares this information with other health care providers.
- Communicates with legislators and/or regulatory agencies regarding epidemiologic issues such as communicable diseases and trauma.
- Participates in the development of nursing measures or procedures that minimize risk factors.

Comprehensive Standard XV — Resource Utilization

Generic Standard The nurse considers factors related to safety, effectiveness, and cost in planning and delivering patient care.

Specialty Standard The emergency nurse collaborates with other health care providers to deliver patient-centered care in a manner consistent with safe, efficient, and cost-effective resource utilization.

Rationale Emergency nurses have the professional responsibility to provide a safe environment and promote appropriate access to care in an efficient, cost-effective manner.

GENERIC MEASUREMENT CRITERIA

1. The nurse evaluates factors related to safety, effectiveness, and cost when two or more practice options would result in the same expected client outcome.
2. The nurse assigns tasks or delegates care based on the needs of the client and the knowledge and skill of the provider selected.
3. The nurse assists the client and significant others in identifying and securing appropriate services available to address health-related needs.

SPECIALTY MEASUREMENT CRITERIA

1. The emergency nurse ensures that requisite supplies and equipment are readily available and an appropriate charge is generated when they are used.

Competent Level

- Ensures that supplies and equipment are readily available and in working order.
- Ensures delivery of efficient and effective care through assessment and evaluation of emergency facility operations.
- Ensures that patient charges are accurate and reflect the care that the patient received.

Excellent Level

- Coordinates appropriate product evaluation.
- Recommends selection and utilization of supplies and equipment.
- Coordinates the maintenance and revision of patient charge systems within the specific department.

2. The emergency nurse takes appropriate measures to optimize the safety of peers, patients, significant others, other health care providers, and self in the emergency care setting.

Competent Level

- Demonstrates knowledge of standardized safety procedures in the emergency care setting.
- Identifies and rectifies sources of potential accidents through daily or periodic inspection.
- Implements safety procedures for each patient in accordance with that patient's specific needs.
- Demonstrates knowledge and compliance with practices that protect the health care provider and reduce the spread of infection in the emergency care setting.
- Demonstrates knowledge and skills necessary to implement the protocol to be followed in the event of an internal or external disaster or threat.
- Recognizes the potential for violence in the emergency setting and institutes appropriate action.

Excellent Level

- Participates in development of policies and procedures related to safety and bloodborne pathogens and Occupational Safety and Health Administration (OSHA) requirements.
- Coordinates education programs related to safety and bloodborne pathogens and OSHA requirements.
- Addresses violence in the emergency setting through the development, implementation, and evaluation of appropriate policies and procedures.
- Educates peers and other health care providers on management of violent situations.
- Participates in community education to increase awareness of violence as a health issue.
- Participates in the development of technology and utilization of products to enhance patient care and safety.

3. The emergency nurse offers medical screening examinations and triages appropriately.

Competent Level

- Promotes access to care through appropriate screening and triage of patients in accordance with COBRA and state guidelines.

Excellent Level

- Participates in the development of policies related to screening examinations and triage.
- Coordinates staff education related to medical screening examinations and triage.

4. The emergency nurse makes staff assignments that reflect acuity, patient needs, and nursing responsibilities, and delegates appropriately to other health care providers.

Competent Level

- Assigns and delegates care that reflects the needs of patients in the department.
- Alerts supervisory personnel to unsafe staffing situations.

Excellent Level

- Adjusts staffing requirements as changes occur in patient volumes, acuity, arrival times, and length of stay.

EMERGENCY
EMERGENCY
EMERGENCY
EMERGENCY
EMERGENCY
EMERGENCY
NURSES**A**SSOCIATION

GLOSSARY

Advanced Life Support (ALS) Interventions for identification and treatment of the patient in a cardiopulmonary crisis. Includes airway management, dysrhythmia recognition and treatment, defibrillation, and pharmacology.

assessment A systematic, dynamic process by which the nurse, through interaction with the client, significant others, and health care providers collects and analyzes data about the client. Data may include the following dimensions: physical, psychological, sociocultural, spiritual, cognitive, functional abilities, developmental, economic, and life-style (ANA, 1991).

Basic Life Support (BLS) Interventions that support breathing and circulation for the patient who is pulseless and breathless. Includes chest compressions and rescue breathing.

certification The process by which a professional is recognized for attainment and application of a specified body of emergency nursing knowledge.

Certified Emergency Nurse (CEN®) A registered professional nurse who has successfully passed the certification examination for emergency nurses. This examination measures attainment and application of a defined body of emergency nursing knowledge needed to function at a competent level.

client Recipient of nursing actions. When the client is an individual, the focus is on the health state, problems, or needs of a single person. When the client is a family or group, the focus is on the health state of the unit as a whole or the reciprocal effects of an individual's health state on the other members of the unit. When the client is a community, the focus is on personal and environmental health and the health risks of population groups. Nursing actions toward clients may be directed to disease or injury prevention, health promotion, health restoration, or health maintenance (ANA, 1991).

collaborative problems An actual or potential health problem that focuses on the pathophysiological response of the body and that nurses are responsible and accountable to identify and treat in collaboration with the physician (Carpenito, 1992).

competent level The level of performance the emergency nurse or an institution should consider in establishing goals for the nurse's professional practice. Each area set forth in the standards does not necessarily have to be met for the nurse's performance to be competent. Competent emergency nursing is demonstrated by sound clinical judgment in autonomous practice.

Consolidated Omnibus Budget Reconciliation Act of 1986 (COBRA) Legislation established to prevent patient dumping due to the lack of monetary resources.

continuity of care An interdisciplinary process that includes clients and significant others in the development of a coordinated plan of care. This process facilitates the client's transition between settings, based on changing needs and available resources (ANA, 1991).

criteria Relevant, measurable indicators of the standards of clinical nursing practice (ANA, 1991).

diagnosis A clinical judgment about the client's response to actual or potential health conditions or needs. Diagnoses provide the basis for determination of a plan of care to achieve expected outcomes (ANA, 1991).

Emergency Nurse Pediatric Course (ENPC) A 16-hour course designed to provide core-level knowledge and psychomotor skills associated with the delivery of professional nursing care to the pediatric patient.

emergency nursing The nursing assessment, diagnosis, and treatment of human responses to actual or potential, sudden or urgent, physical or psychosocial problems that are primarily episodic and acute in nature.

entry level into practice The level of competence necessary for a nurse to begin practicing. It includes a registered nurse who is competent in basic nursing assessment and interventions, but who continues to develop skills and expertise, and develops knowledge-based judgments through experience and education.

evaluation The process of determining both the patient's progress toward the attainment of expected outcomes and the effectiveness of nursing care (ANA, 1991).

excellent level Practice that surpasses the competent level and contributes to the growth of emergency nursing practice.

generic standards Standards that apply to the care that is provided to all clients and apply to all registered nurses engaged in clinical practice, regardless of clinical specialty, practice setting, or educational preparation (ANA, 1991).

guidelines Description of a process of client care management that has the potential for improving the quality of clinical and consumer decision making. Guidelines are systematically developed statements based on available scientific evidence and expert opinion (ANA, 1991).

health care providers Individuals with special expertise who provide health care services or assistance to clients. They may include nurses, physicians, paramedics, first responders, psychologists, social workers, nutritionists and dieticians, and various therapists. Providers also may include service organizations and vendors (ANA, 1991).

implementation May include any or all of these activities: intervening, delegating, coordinating. The client, significant others, or health care providers may be designated to implement interventions within the plan of care (ANA, 1991).

nursing The diagnosis and treatment of human responses to actual or potential health problems (ANA, 1980).

nursing diagnosis A clinical judgment about individual, family, or community responses to actual or potential health problems or life processes. Nursing diagnoses provide the basis for selection of nursing interventions to achieve outcomes for which the nurse is accountable (Carpenito, 1992).

Occupational Safety and Health Administration (OSHA) A federal regulatory agency established to promote safety in the workplace through mandated guidelines.

outcome identification Measurable, expected, client-focused goals as identified by the nurse through collaboration with the client and health care providers, when possible (ANA, 1991).

patient A person who is ill or injured and in a position to receive health care.

Pediatric Advanced Life Support (PALS) A 12-hour course to provide knowledge and skills for identification and management for cardiopulmonary emergencies in the neonate and pediatric patient. Includes airway management, dysrhythmia recognition and treatment, defibrillation, venous access, and pharmacology.

plan of care Comprehensive outline of care to be delivered to attain expected outcomes (ANA, 1991).

rationale Provides the justification for the standard.

significant others Family members, parents, caregivers, and/or those significant to the patient.

specialty standards Standards that apply to all nurses practicing within a specific specialty setting. Specialty standards in this document apply to emergency care settings.

standard Authoritative statement enunciated and promulgated by the profession and by which the quality of practice, service, or education can be judged (ANA, 1991).

Standards of Care Authoritative statements that describe a competent level of clinical nursing practice demonstrated through assessment, diagnosis, outcome identification, planning, implementation, and evaluation (ANA, 1991).

Standards of Professional Performance Authoritative statements that describe competent level of behavior in the professional role, including activities related to quality of care, performance appraisal, education, collegiality, ethics, collaboration, research, and resource utilization (ANA, 1991).

Trauma Nursing Core Course (TNCC) A 16- or 20-hour course designed to provide core-level trauma knowledge and psychomotor skills associated with the delivery of professional nursing care to the trauma patient.

triage The process by which patients are evaluated and classified according to the type and urgency of their condition, for the purpose of determining treatment priorities. Patients are identified promptly using rapid assessments and interventions to maintain the patient flow through the emergency department and provide information and referrals and to allay anxieties of patients and significant others.

EMERGENCY
EMERGENCY
EMERGENCY
EMERGENCY
EMERGENCY
EMERGENCY
NURSES**A**SSOCIATION

RESOURCES

American Heart Association. (1987). *Textbook of advanced cardiac life support* (2nd ed.). Dallas, TX: Author.

American Heart Association. (1988). *Textbook of pediatric advanced life support*. Dallas, TX: Author.

American Heart Association. (1992). *Cardiopulmonary resuscitation—basic rescuer course*. Dallas, TX: Author.

American Hospital Association. (1992). *A patient's bill of rights* (cat. no. 157759). Chicago, IL: Author.

American Medical Association. (1992). Guidelines for cardiopulmonary resuscitation and emergency cardiac care. *Journal of the American Medical Association*. 268 (16), 2171.

American Nurses Association. (1980). *Nursing: A social policy statement*. Kansas City, MO: Author.

American Nurses Association. (1985). *Code for nurses with interpretive statements*. Kansas City, MO: Author.

American Nurses Association. (1991). *Standards of clinical nursing practice*. Kansas City, MO: Author.

Carpenito, Lynda Juall. (1992). *Nursing diagnosis—application to clinical practice* (4th ed.). Philadelphia, PA: J.B. Lippincott Co.

Consolidated Omnibus Budget Reconciliation Act of 1986, 42 U.S.C.A. § 1395dd (1993).

Emergency Nurses Association. (1989). *Code of ethics for emergency nurses with interpretive statements*. Chicago, IL: Author.

Emergency Nurses Association. (1990). *Emergency department patient classification systems manual*. Chicago, IL: Author.

Emergency Nurses Association. (1991). *Emergency clinical nurse specialist guidelines*. Chicago, IL: Author.

Emergency Nurses Association. (1991). *Legislative manual.* Chicago, IL: Author.

Emergency Nurses Association. (1991). Position statement: Autonomous emergency nursing practice. *ENA position statements* (pp. 7-8). Park Ridge, IL: Author.

Emergency Nurses Association. (1991). Position statement: CEN credentialing and review courses. *ENA position statements* (pp. 13-14). Park Ridge, IL: Author.

Emergency Nurses Association. (1991). Position statement: Telephone advice. *ENA position statements* (pp. 85-86). Park Ridge, IL: Author.

Emergency Nurses Association. (1991). *Trauma nursing core course.* (3rd ed.). Park Ridge, IL: Author.

Emergency Nurses Association. (1992). Position statement: Injury prevention. *ENA position statements* (pp. 35-47). Park Ridge, IL: Author.

Emergency Nurses Association. (1992). Position statement: Resuscitative decisions. *ENA position statements* (pp. 63-64). Park Ridge, IL: Author.

Emergency Nurses Association. (1992). *Emergency nurses guide to nursing diagnosis.* Park Ridge, IL: Author.

Emergency Nurses Association. (1992). Position statement: Integration of emergency nursing concepts in nursing curricula. *ENA position statements* (pp. 49). Park Ridge, IL: Author.

Emergency Nurses Association. (1992). *Triage: Meeting the challenge.* Park Ridge, IL: Author.

Emergency Nurses Association. (1993). *About your emergency care—your visit to the emergency department: what to expect.* Park Ridge, IL: Author.

Emergency Nurses Association. (1993). *Emergency nursing core curriculum* (4th ed.). Philadelphia, PA: W.B. Saunders.

Emergency Nurses Association. (1993). *Emergency nursing pediatric course.* Park Ridge, IL: Author.

Emergency Nurses Association. (1993). [Graduate programs offering emergency- or trauma-related nursing tracks]. Unpublished raw data.

Emergency Nurses Association. (1993). *Orientation to emergency nursing: Diversity in practice.* Park Ridge, IL: Author.

Emergency Nurses Association. (1993). *Pediatric emergency nursing resource guide.* Park Ridge, IL: Author.

Emergency Nurses Association. (1993). Position statement: Access to care. *ENA position statements* (pp. 1-3). Park Ridge, IL: Author.

Emergency Nurses Association. (1993). Position statement: Advanced practice in emergency nursing. *ENA position statements* (pp. 5-6). Park Ridge, IL: Author.

Emergency Nurses Association. (1993). Position statement: Bloodborne infectious diseases. *ENA position statements* (pp. 9-12). Park Ridge, IL: Author.

Emergency Nurses Association. (1993). Position statement: Chemical impairment of emergency nurses. *ENA position statements* (pp. 15-16). Park Ridge, IL: Author.

Emergency Nurses Association. (1993). Position statement: Collaborative research. *ENA position statements* (pp. 19-20). Park Ridge, IL: Author.

Emergency Nurses Association. (1993). Position statement: Conscious sedation. *ENA position statements* (pp. 19-20). Park Ridge, IL: Author.

Emergency Nurses Association. (1993). Position statement: Enhanced 9-1-1 systems. *ENA position statements* (pp. 21-22). Park Ridge, IL: Author.

Emergency Nurses Association. (1993). Position statement: Hepatitis B immunization for emergency nursing personnel. *ENA position statements* (pp. 23-24). Park Ridge, IL: Author.

Emergency Nurses Association. (1993). Position statement: Hospital and emergency department overcrowding. *ENA position statements* (pp. 27-30). Park Ridge, IL: Author.

Emergency Nurses Association. (1993). Position statement: Human neglect and abuse. *ENA position statements* (pp. 27-29). Park Ridge, IL: Author.

Emergency Nurses Association. (1993). Position statement: Impact of nursing shortage. *ENA position statements* (pp. 31-33). Park Ridge, IL: Author.

Emergency Nurses Association. (1993). Position statement: Interfacility transport of the critically ill or injured patient. *ENA position statements* (pp. 51-52). Park Ridge, IL: Author.

Emergency Nurses Association. (1993). Position statement: Observation/holding areas. *ENA position statements* (pp. 55-56). Park Ridge, IL: Author.

Emergency Nurses Association. (1993). Position statement: Protection of animal subjects. *ENA position statements* (pp. 59-60). Park Ridge, IL: Author.

Emergency Nurses Association. (1993). Position statement: Protection of human subjects' rights. *ENA position statements* (pp. 61-62). Park Ridge, IL: Author.

Emergency Nurses Association. (1993). Position statement: Role of the emergency nurse in the education of the prehospital care provider. *ENA position statements* (pp. 65-66). Park Ridge, IL: Author.

Emergency Nurses Association. (1993). Position statement: Role of the emergency nurse in tissue and organ procurement. *ENA position statements* (pp. 67-68). Park Ridge, IL: Author.

Emergency Nurses Association. (1993). Position statement: Role of the registered nurse in the prehospital environment. *ENA position statements* (pp. 69-72). Park Ridge, IL: Author.

Emergency Nurses Association. (1993). Position statement: Staffing and productivity in the emergency care setting. *ENA position statements* (pp. 75-76). Park Ridge, IL: Author.

Emergency Nurses Association. (1993). Position statement: Stress management. *ENA position statements* (pp. 79-80). Park Ridge, IL: Author.

Emergency Nurses Association. (1993). Position statement: Substance abuse. *ENA position statements* (pp. 81-84). Park Ridge, IL: Author.

Emergency Nurses Association. (1993). Position statement: Treatment of sexual assault survivors. *ENA position statements* (pp. 87-89). Park Ridge, IL: Author.

Emergency Nurses Association. (1993). Position statement: Use of non-registered (non-RN) caregivers in emergency care. *ENA position statements* (pp. 93-94). Park Ridge, IL: Author.

Emergency Nurses Association. (1993). Position statement: Violence in the emergency setting. *ENA position statements* (pp. 99-101). Park Ridge, IL: Author.

Emergency Nurses Association. (1993). *Research initiatives.* Park Ridge, IL: Author.

Joint Commission on Accreditation of Healthcare Organizations. (1992). *Accreditation manual for hospitals, 1993, volume 1, Standards.* Oakbrook Terrace, IL: Author.

Occupational Safety and Health Administration, 29 C.F.R. § 1910.1030 (1992).